This Biking Book Belongs To:

_____

_____

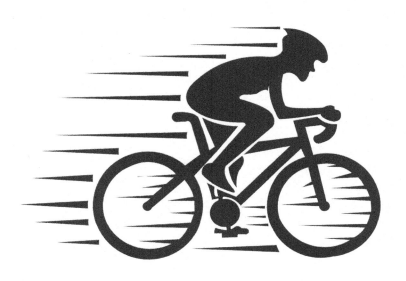

Riding Trail: _____

Location: _____

Date: _____ Distance_____

Companions: _____

Weather

Temperature:_____

Trail Difficulty

1   2   3   4   5

Thoughts About This Ride

_____

_____

_____

_____

_____

_____

_____

_____

Overall Rating ☆ ☆ ☆ ☆ ☆

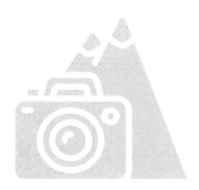

Notes – Memories - Photos

Riding Trail: _____

Location: _____

Date: _____ Distance_____

Companions: _____

Weather

Temperature:_____

Trail Difficulty

1   2   3   4   5

Thoughts About This Ride

_____
_____
_____
_____
_____
_____
_____
_____
_____

Overall Rating ☆ ☆ ☆ ☆ ☆

Notes – Memories - Photos

Riding Trail: _____

Location: _____

Date: _____   Distance_____

Companions: _____

Weather

Temperature:_____

Trail Difficulty

1   2   3   4   5

Thoughts About This Ride

_____
_____
_____
_____
_____
_____
_____
_____
_____

Overall Rating   ☆ ☆ ☆ ☆ ☆

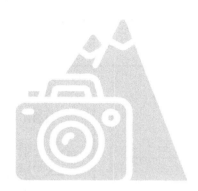

Notes – Memories - Photos

Riding Trail: _____

Location: _____

Date: _____   Distance_____

Companions: _____

Weather

Temperature:_____

Trail Difficulty

1   2   3   4   5

Thoughts About This Ride

_____
_____
_____
_____
_____
_____
_____
_____

Overall Rating   ☆ ☆ ☆ ☆ ☆

Notes – Memories - Photos

Riding Trail: _____

Location: _____

Date: _____   Distance_____

Companions: _____

Weather

Temperature:_____

Trail Difficulty

1   2   3   4   5

Thoughts About This Ride

_____
_____
_____
_____
_____
_____
_____
_____

Overall Rating   ☆ ☆ ☆ ☆ ☆

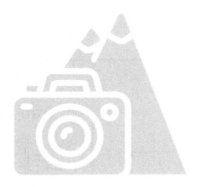

Notes – Memories - Photos

Riding Trail: _____

Location: _____

Date: _____ Distance_____

Companions: _____

Weather

Temperature:_____

Trail Difficulty

1 2 3 4 5

Thoughts About This Ride

_____

_____

_____

_____

_____

_____

_____

_____

Overall Rating ☆ ☆ ☆ ☆ ☆

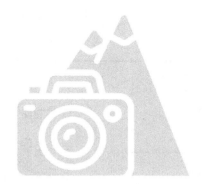

Notes – Memories - Photos

Riding Trail: _____

Location: _____

Date: _____ Distance_____

Companions: _____

Weather

Temperature:_____

Trail Difficulty

1   2   3   4   5

Thoughts About This Ride

_____
_____
_____
_____
_____
_____
_____
_____

Overall Rating ☆ ☆ ☆ ☆ ☆

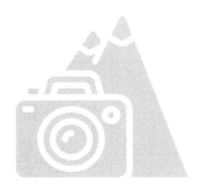

Notes – Memories - Photos

Riding Trail: _____

Location: _____

Date: _____ Distance_____

Companions: _____

Weather

Temperature:_____

Trail Difficulty

1   2   3   4   5

Thoughts About This Ride

_____
_____
_____
_____
_____
_____
_____
_____
_____

Overall Rating ☆ ☆ ☆ ☆ ☆

Notes – Memories - Photos

Riding Trail: _____

Location: _____

Date: _____ Distance_____

Companions: _____

Weather

Temperature:_____

Trail Difficulty

1   2   3   4   5

Thoughts About This Ride

_____
_____
_____
_____
_____
_____
_____
_____

Overall Rating ☆ ☆ ☆ ☆ ☆

Notes – Memories - Photos

Riding Trail: _____

Location: _____

Date: _____ Distance_____

Companions: _____

Weather

Temperature:_____

Trail Difficulty

1   2   3   4   5

Thoughts About This Ride

_____
_____
_____
_____
_____
_____
_____
_____

Overall Rating   ☆ ☆ ☆ ☆ ☆

Notes – Memories - Photos

Riding Trail: _____

Location: _____

Date: _____ Distance_____

Companions: _____

Weather

Temperature:_____

Trail Difficulty

1   2   3   4   5

Thoughts About This Ride

_____

_____

_____

_____

_____

_____

_____

_____

Overall Rating ☆ ☆ ☆ ☆ ☆

Notes – Memories - Photos

Riding Trail: _____

Location: _____

Date: _____ Distance_____

Companions: _____

Weather

Temperature:_____

Trail Difficulty

1   2   3   4   5

Thoughts About This Ride

_____
_____
_____
_____
_____
_____
_____
_____

Overall Rating ☆ ☆ ☆ ☆ ☆

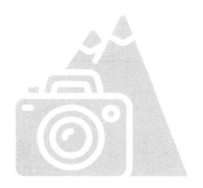

Notes – Memories - Photos

Riding Trail: _____

Location: _____

Date: _____ Distance_____

Companions: _____

Weather

Temperature:_____

Trail Difficulty

1   2   3   4   5

Thoughts About This Ride

_____

_____

_____

_____

_____

_____

_____

_____

_____

Overall Rating ☆ ☆ ☆ ☆ ☆

Notes – Memories - Photos

Riding Trail: _____

Location: _____

Date: _____ Distance_____

Companions: _____

Weather

Temperature:_____

Trail Difficulty

1   2   3   4   5

Thoughts About This Ride

_____

_____

_____

_____

_____

_____

_____

_____

_____

Overall Rating ☆ ☆ ☆ ☆ ☆

Notes – Memories - Photos

Riding Trail: _____

Location: _____

Date: _____ Distance_____

Companions: _____

Weather

Temperature:_____

Trail Difficulty

1   2   3   4   5

Thoughts About This Ride

_____
_____
_____
_____
_____
_____
_____
_____

Overall Rating ☆ ☆ ☆ ☆ ☆

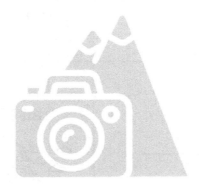

Notes – Memories - Photos

Riding Trail: _____

Location: _____

Date: _____   Distance_____

Companions: _____

Weather

Temperature:_____

Trail Difficulty

1   2   3   4   5

Thoughts About This Ride

_____
_____
_____
_____
_____
_____
_____
_____

Overall Rating ☆ ☆ ☆ ☆ ☆

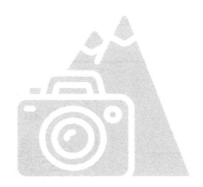

Notes – Memories - Photos

Riding Trail: _____

Location: _____

Date: _____ Distance_____

Companions: _____

Weather

Temperature:_____

Trail Difficulty

1   2   3   4   5

Thoughts About This Ride

_____
_____
_____
_____
_____
_____
_____
_____

Overall Rating ☆ ☆ ☆ ☆ ☆

Notes – Memories - Photos

Riding Trail: _____

Location: _____

Date: _____ Distance_____

Companions: _____

Weather

Temperature:_____

Trail Difficulty

1   2   3   4   5

Thoughts About This Ride

_____

_____

_____

_____

_____

_____

_____

_____

Overall Rating ☆ ☆ ☆ ☆ ☆

Notes – Memories - Photos

Riding Trail: _____

Location: _____

Date: _____ Distance_____

Companions: _____

Weather

Temperature:_____

Trail Difficulty

1   2   3   4   5

Thoughts About This Ride

_____
_____
_____
_____
_____
_____
_____
_____

Overall Rating ☆ ☆ ☆ ☆ ☆

Notes – Memories - Photos

Riding Trail: _____

Location: _____

Date: _____ Distance_____

Companions: _____

Weather

Temperature:_____

Trail Difficulty

1   2   3   4   5

Thoughts About This Ride

_____
_____
_____
_____
_____
_____
_____
_____

Overall Rating ☆ ☆ ☆ ☆ ☆

Notes – Memories - Photos

Riding Trail: _____

Location: _____

Date: _____ Distance_____

Companions: _____

Weather

Temperature:_____

Trail Difficulty

1   2   3   4   5

Thoughts About This Ride

_____
_____
_____
_____
_____
_____
_____
_____

Overall Rating ☆ ☆ ☆ ☆ ☆

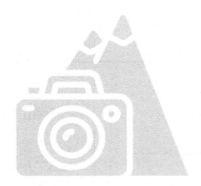

Notes – Memories - Photos

Riding Trail: _____

Location: _____

Date: _____ Distance_____

Companions: _____

Weather

Temperature:_____

Trail Difficulty

1   2   3   4   5

Thoughts About This Ride

_____

_____

_____

_____

_____

_____

_____

_____

_____

Overall Rating ☆ ☆ ☆ ☆ ☆

Notes – Memories - Photos

Riding Trail: _____

Location: _____

Date: _____ Distance_____

Companions: _____

Weather

Temperature:_____

Trail Difficulty

1   2   3   4   5

Thoughts About This Ride

_____
_____
_____
_____
_____
_____
_____
_____

Overall Rating ☆ ☆ ☆ ☆ ☆

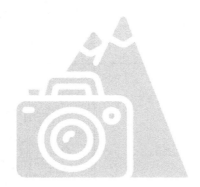

Notes – Memories - Photos

Riding Trail: _____

Location: _____

Date: _____   Distance_____

Companions: _____

Weather

Temperature:_____

Trail Difficulty

1   2   3   4   5

Thoughts About This Ride

_____

_____

_____

_____

_____

_____

_____

_____

Overall Rating ☆ ☆ ☆ ☆ ☆

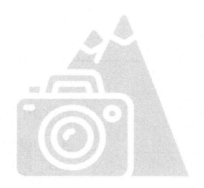

Notes – Memories - Photos

Riding Trail: _____

Location: _____

Date: _____ Distance_____

Companions: _____

Weather

Temperature:_____

Trail Difficulty

1   2   3   4   5

Thoughts About This Ride

_____
_____
_____
_____
_____
_____
_____
_____

Overall Rating ☆ ☆ ☆ ☆ ☆

Notes – Memories - Photos

Riding Trail: _____

Location: _____

Date: _____ Distance_____

Companions: _____

Weather

Temperature:_____

Trail Difficulty

1   2   3   4   5

Thoughts About This Ride

_____
_____
_____
_____
_____
_____
_____
_____

Overall Rating ☆ ☆ ☆ ☆ ☆

Notes – Memories - Photos

Riding Trail: _____

Location: _____

Date: _____ Distance_____

Companions: _____

Weather

Temperature:_____

Trail Difficulty

1   2   3   4   5

Thoughts About This Ride

_____

_____

_____

_____

_____

_____

_____

_____

Overall Rating ☆ ☆ ☆ ☆ ☆

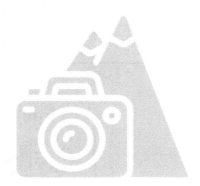

Notes – Memories - Photos

Riding Trail: _____

Location: _____

Date: _____ Distance_____

Companions: _____

Weather

Temperature:_____

Trail Difficulty

1   2   3   4   5

Thoughts About This Ride

_____
_____
_____
_____
_____
_____
_____
_____

Overall Rating ☆ ☆ ☆ ☆ ☆

Notes – Memories - Photos

Riding Trail: _____

Location: _____

Date: _____   Distance_____

Companions: _____

Weather

Temperature:_____

Trail Difficulty

1   2   3   4   5

Thoughts About This Ride

_____
_____
_____
_____
_____
_____
_____
_____

Overall Rating ☆ ☆ ☆ ☆ ☆

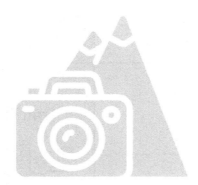

Notes – Memories - Photos

Riding Trail: _____

Location: _____

Date: _____ Distance_____

Companions: _____

Weather

Temperature:_____

Trail Difficulty

1   2   3   4   5

Thoughts About This Ride

_____
_____
_____
_____
_____
_____
_____
_____

Overall Rating ☆ ☆ ☆ ☆ ☆

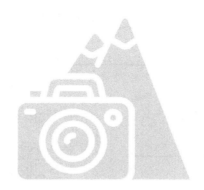

Notes – Memories - Photos

Riding Trail: _____

Location: _____

Date: _____ Distance_____

Companions: _____

Weather

Temperature:_____

Trail Difficulty

1   2   3   4   5

Thoughts About This Ride

_____
_____
_____
_____
_____
_____
_____
_____

Overall Rating ☆ ☆ ☆ ☆ ☆

Notes – Memories - Photos

Riding Trail: _____

Location: _____

Date: _____ Distance_____

Companions: _____

Weather

Temperature:_____

Trail Difficulty

1   2   3   4   5

Thoughts About This Ride

_____

_____

_____

_____

_____

_____

_____

_____

Overall Rating ☆ ☆ ☆ ☆ ☆

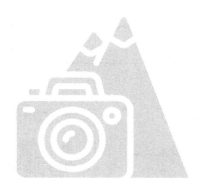

Notes – Memories - Photos

Riding Trail: _____

Location: _____

Date: _____ Distance_____

Companions: _____

Weather

Temperature:_____

Trail Difficulty

1   2   3   4   5

Thoughts About This Ride

_____

_____

_____

_____

_____

_____

_____

_____

Overall Rating   ☆ ☆ ☆ ☆ ☆

Notes – Memories - Photos

Riding Trail: _____

Location: _____

Date: _____ Distance_____

Companions: _____

Weather

Temperature:_____

Trail Difficulty

1   2   3   4   5

Thoughts About This Ride

_____
_____
_____
_____
_____
_____
_____
_____

Overall Rating   ☆ ☆ ☆ ☆ ☆

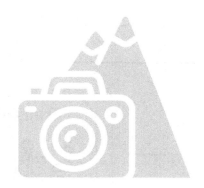

Notes – Memories - Photos

Riding Trail: _____

Location: _____

Date: _____ Distance_____

Companions: _____

Weather

Temperature:_____

Trail Difficulty

1   2   3   4   5

Thoughts About This Ride

_____

_____

_____

_____

_____

_____

_____

_____

Overall Rating   ☆ ☆ ☆ ☆ ☆

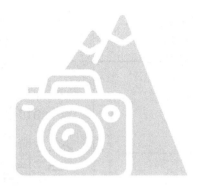

Notes – Memories - Photos

Riding Trail: _____

Location: _____

Date: _____ Distance_____

Companions: _____

Weather

Temperature:_____

Trail Difficulty

1   2   3   4   5

Thoughts About This Ride

_____
_____
_____
_____
_____
_____
_____
_____

Overall Rating ☆ ☆ ☆ ☆ ☆

Notes – Memories - Photos

Riding Trail: _____

Location: _____

Date: _____ Distance_____

Companions: _____

Weather	Trail Difficulty
Temperature:_____	
☀ ⛅ ☁ 🌧	1 2 3 4 5

Thoughts About This Ride

_____

_____

_____

_____

_____

_____

_____

_____

Overall Rating ☆ ☆ ☆ ☆ ☆

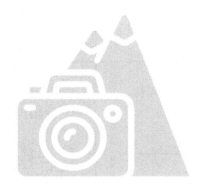

Notes – Memories - Photos

Riding Trail: _____

Location: _____

Date: _____ Distance_____

Companions: _____

Weather

Temperature:_____

Trail Difficulty

1   2   3   4   5

Thoughts About This Ride

_____
_____
_____
_____
_____
_____
_____
_____

Overall Rating ☆ ☆ ☆ ☆ ☆

Notes – Memories - Photos

Riding Trail: _____

Location: _____

Date: _____ Distance_____

Companions: _____

Weather

Temperature:_____

Trail Difficulty

1   2   3   4   5

Thoughts About This Ride

_____
_____
_____
_____
_____
_____
_____
_____

Overall Rating ☆ ☆ ☆ ☆ ☆

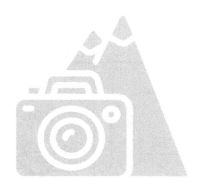

Notes – Memories - Photos

Riding Trail: _____

Location: _____

Date: _____ Distance_____

Companions: _____

Weather

Temperature:_____

Trail Difficulty

1   2   3   4   5

Thoughts About This Ride

_____
_____
_____
_____
_____
_____
_____
_____

Overall Rating ☆ ☆ ☆ ☆ ☆

Notes – Memories - Photos

Riding Trail: _____

Location: _____

Date: _____   Distance_____

Companions: _____

Weather

Temperature:_____

Trail Difficulty

1   2   3   4   5

Thoughts About This Ride

_____
_____
_____
_____
_____
_____
_____
_____

Overall Rating   ☆ ☆ ☆ ☆ ☆

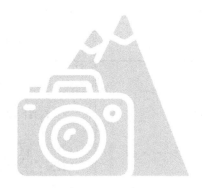

Notes – Memories - Photos

Riding Trail: _____

Location: _____

Date: _____ Distance_____

Companions: _____

Weather

Temperature:_____

Trail Difficulty

1   2   3   4   5

Thoughts About This Ride

_____
_____
_____
_____
_____
_____
_____
_____

Overall Rating ☆ ☆ ☆ ☆ ☆

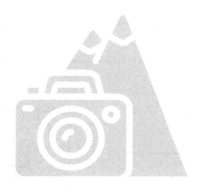

Notes – Memories - Photos

Riding Trail: _____

Location: _____

Date: _____ Distance_____

Companions: _____

Weather

Temperature:_____

Trail Difficulty

1   2   3   4   5

Thoughts About This Ride

_____
_____
_____
_____
_____
_____
_____
_____

Overall Rating   ☆ ☆ ☆ ☆ ☆

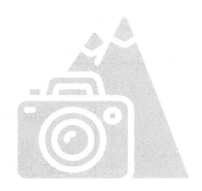

Notes – Memories - Photos

Riding Trail: _____

Location: _____

Date: _____ Distance_____

Companions: _____

Weather

Temperature:_____

Trail Difficulty

1   2   3   4   5

Thoughts About This Ride

_____

_____

_____

_____

_____

_____

_____

_____

Overall Rating ☆ ☆ ☆ ☆ ☆

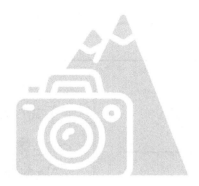

Notes – Memories - Photos

Riding Trail: _____

Location: _____

Date: _____   Distance_____

Companions: _____

Weather

Temperature:_____

Trail Difficulty

1   2   3   4   5

Thoughts About This Ride

_____
_____
_____
_____
_____
_____
_____
_____

Overall Rating   ☆ ☆ ☆ ☆ ☆

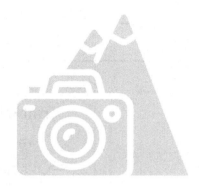

Notes – Memories - Photos

Riding Trail: _____

Location: _____

Date: _____ Distance_____

Companions: _____

Weather

Temperature:_____

Trail Difficulty

1   2   3   4   5

Thoughts About This Ride

_____

_____

_____

_____

_____

_____

_____

_____

Overall Rating ☆ ☆ ☆ ☆ ☆

Notes – Memories - Photos

Riding Trail: _____

Location: _____

Date: _____   Distance_____

Companions: _____

Weather

Temperature:_____

Trail Difficulty

1   2   3   4   5

Thoughts About This Ride

_____
_____
_____
_____
_____
_____
_____
_____

Overall Rating   ☆ ☆ ☆ ☆ ☆

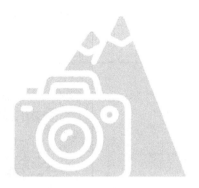

Notes – Memories - Photos

Riding Trail: _____

Location: _____

Date: _____   Distance_____

Companions: _____

Weather

Temperature:_____

Trail Difficulty

1   2   3   4   5

Thoughts About This Ride

_____
_____
_____
_____
_____
_____
_____
_____

Overall Rating   ☆ ☆ ☆ ☆ ☆

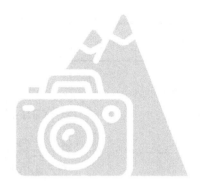

Notes – Memories - Photos

Riding Trail: _____

Location: _____

Date: _____ Distance_____

Companions: _____

Weather

Temperature:_____

Trail Difficulty

1   2   3   4   5

Thoughts About This Ride

_____
_____
_____
_____
_____
_____
_____
_____

Overall Rating ☆ ☆ ☆ ☆ ☆

Notes – Memories - Photos

Riding Trail: _____

Location: _____

Date: _____ Distance_____

Companions: _____

Weather

Temperature:_____

Trail Difficulty

1   2   3   4   5

Thoughts About This Ride

_____

_____

_____

_____

_____

_____

_____

_____

Overall Rating   ☆ ☆ ☆ ☆ ☆

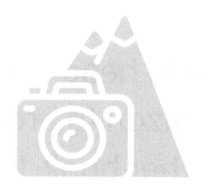

Notes – Memories - Photos

Time to head back to Amazon to order another book. If you enjoyed this
log book, we hope you will share your opinion by leaving a review on Amazon.
Thank you,
Wandering Trails

Made in the USA
Monee, IL
08 December 2021

84303695R00059